'

My LifePlan®

'Life Plan'/
'Life Coaching'

'Life Plan'

Dear Sir/Ms,

This Life Plan is based upon some of the skills and knowledge, understanding and wisdom I've gained across my journey of life so far. These are just some ideas and suggestions and nothing else and hopefully are of benefit to yourselves and the people you come across. I've kept the areas broad, and objectives/goals general, so people can take from this what is suited and relevant to them. You may need or want some, all or none of this Life Plan. **If you can take something from this Life Plan, it is to live a better, healthier life, and come back to the house, your home, in Heaven/Paradise.** All I ask is to have a read and decide for yourself.

Objectives/Goals
- Be more fit, healthy, relaxed, content and happy.
- Some time for people in your life.
- Simplify life in general.
- Increase spiritual-religious life, including charity work.
- Help yourself, and your family and friends, be more financially sound to do the things they would like to do in their life.
- Work part-time, casual or volunteer in certain area to free up time to do the things that are important, and you want to do, in your life.
- Take up some hobbies and interests

Life Plan areas
1. Health
2. Activities
3. Faith
4. Relationships

Action Plan
1.   Health
- *Goal*: Be more fit, healthy, relaxed, content and happy.

- *Diet*
  → There is a wise saying, 'Let Food by thy Medicine'. This is especially when combined with other areas of health like, Exercise, Therapy and Stress Management, Personal Development and Image/Presentation/Personal Hygiene.

  →Diet is usually a combination of 'Protein', 'Carbohydrates' and 'Fats'

  Protein - Soy, Eggs, Fish/Tins of Tuna, Chicken, Beef, Lamb, Protein-Shake;

Carbohydrate – Fruit and Vegetables (there is a plethora of fruits and vegetables which are healthy and delicious); Rice – Basmati less fatty than Jasmine, pasta, Baked Beans, Lentils, Cereal (I prefer Oats or Muesli with Fruit – E.g. Sun Sol or Lowan at Woolworths, or ALDI, or Coles), LSA powder, Multi-Fibre Powder Drink (E.g. Networking companies, like, Nutriway, Isagenix, GNLD).

Fats - Fish oils; Olive Oil; Avocado; Mixed nuts, e.g. from Markets - Walnut, Almond, Cashew, Macadamia, Pistaschio, Corn chip.

→ If a person wants to maximize their diet and or if they feel they get enough nutrition from their diets, and do not want to take supplements, vitamins and minerals, then I recommend two devices:

Nutri-Bullet (as advertised on TVSN/TV Shopping Network)
This is a high-powered blender that can blend almost anything in the form of fruit and vegetables, from Greens (Spinach, Celery, Kale, Broccoli, Cucumber, Zucchini) and Berries (strawberries, blackberries, blueberries), Citrus Fruits (Orange, Mandarin, Tomato and Kiwi Fruit) and other fruit and vegetables like carrots, bananas and apples.

You can add a banana and cereal, especially muesli or oats, to thicken the mixture and make it sweeter and better tasting. Also add some water or milk to turn the ingredients into a puree or to water it down.

For a slimmer/lean person, and or person with acid in their bodies, I would emphasize 'Green Vegetables'. For a fatter/obese person, some citrus-berry fruits can help stimulate movement and activity and lose weight.

Soup Mate Pro/Soup Maker – Seven Day Soup Diet (as advertised on TVSN/TV Shopping Network)

Inventor and entrepreneur, Brendan McCarthy, came up with a blender similar to Nutri-Bullet, the Soup Mate Pro. It is a 10-in-one blender. It not only blends the ingredients, it also cooks it and turns into a consistent puree. The Soup Mate Pro is fantastic for becoming healthy, losing weight and fighting off diseases and illnesses. It is a fantastic device to have for people with sicknesses, diseases or illnesses, and especially as a form of prevention.

- **Supplements**
  → **Mainly Protein-Shake or Multi-Vitamin, Anti-oxidants, Fish Oils, Olive Oil and Probiotics**
  → Vitamins and Supplements are concentrated food and medicine. They have proper quantities and qualities of ingredients, whereas standard food is not measured and examined enough. You may reach old age with no proper diet

and supplements, but then again you may not; the risk is too much for one's health and wellbeing.

→ Protein-Shake (either high in Protein to keep healthy weight or Protein-Carbohydrate as a meal replacement; has plenty of vitamins. Networking companies are very good for Protein Shakes, like, Nutriway, Isagenix, GNLD, USANA). Fills in the gaps of your diet and lifestyle.

→ Multi-vitamin (Nutriway - Double X and Daily, Isagenix, GNLD, Swisse, Centrum) – Fills in the gaps of your diet and lifestyle. Make sure the Multi-Vitamin does not clash with other supplements, medications and food, possibly causing dangerous chemical reactions. You can either consume a Multi-Vitamin every day, every few days or once a week, in combination with say a Protein-Shake.

→ Anti-oxidants – helps control or get rid of free radicals/bad chemicals in your body. Vitamins A, B, C, D, E. Carotenoids (Vitamin A) are a good combination with Vitamins C and E. Good to have a system or program of vitamins and anti-oxidants, instead of bits and pieces, which is really hit and miss and not as effective.

- There are Economy Packs from Chemists, like Chemist Warehouse and Vitamin King, and Networking companies.
- *Vitamin A* – Pumpkin, Carrots, Capsicum, Nectarines, Peaches, Plums and Sweet Potato; *Vitamin C* - Oranges, Mandarins, Kiwi fruit, Lemon and Lime; *Vitamin E* – Greens like Peas, Beans, Spinach, Broccoli, Cucumber, Zucchini.

→ Fish Oils (Omega-3)/Olive Oil. – helps the brain, heart, eyes, cholesterol, cleans arteries, arthritis and joints. Economy Pack from Chemist. I recommend going for 1500mg with more EPA and DHA, for example Swisse (red and white container) and Caruso.

→ Olive Oil - Olive Oil is similar to Fish Oils, as an anti-oxidant, and is more linked to Vitamin E. People can have a few direct eating/tablespoons of Olive Oil.

→ Probiotics – According to research, in general 20-25 billion good bacteria is needed to make a good probiotic. Poor probiotics are lost in the acid of the stomach before they even reach the intestines. A good probiotic and its good bacteria will reach the intestines and have a stronger and positive effect. The stomach and intestines are classed as the second brain, as a lot of our time is spent consuming food and beverages, and a large quantity of serotonin, the happy chemical in our brain, comes from the stomach.

→ There are side vitamins and minerals a person may lack in:

Calcium-Magnesium & Vitamin D: For nerves, muscle and bones. Relaxation and Stress Management. Most people are usually low in Vitamin D, which can be gained from Sunlight and the tablet form. Examples are Networking company, GNLD 'Cal-Mag' (with Vitamin D).

Glucosomine, including Condriton:
Fantastic for aches and pains. Most brands are usually good, especially the Networking companies like Nutriway-Amway, Isagenix/GNLD/Jeunesse and USANA.

Zinc: Good for mind and body, immune system, skin and sexual/reproductive health. When under stress, some people get depleted in the mineral of Zinc. Zinc also helps keep the walls of the arteries in your body elastic.

Silica: For Nails, Hair and Skin, especially Skin as muscles are also made of skin.

Powders: The *Bioglan/Nature's Way* brands at, Chemists and some Supermarkets, are powdered supplements of different varieties – Chia Seeds, Cacao, Camu, Brown Rice, Greens, Beetroot, Kale and Acai.

→ You can take specific supplements if certain things are needed or missing in your body, for example:

- Cereal: Good to give positive mood and feeling, not just fibre, for e.g. Muesli. People usually have Cereal in the morning before a busy day, lasting until lunch or even all the way to dinner; Cereal is that powerful. Cereal can also be used as a snack throughout the day.

- Metamucil/Cleanse-Detox (powder): For fibre, detox/losing weight and cholesterol.

• *Exercise*
I can't emphasize the significant effects of exercise on your health, for keeping fit, stress management and remaining positive. All you need is 20-30 minutes a day, or 10 minutes a day at minimum.
→ Stretching: From Head to Toe.
→ Cardio/Walking/Jogging: Light-to-Moderate cardio is usually recommended, or harder-intense for other people.
→ Gym: You can join a gym and a few days a week or everyday. There can be a blend of Cardio (Treadmill, Cross-Trainer, Rowing Machine and Exercise Bike), and Weights-Strengthening (training one or some body parts)
→ Exercise Equipment at home: This can provide an alternative to going to the gym, or if you do not feel like going to the gym, stressed or sick. You can buy, from a fitness store, a treadmill, small exercise bike or rowing machine → Strengthening: With a stretch, some good strengthening techniques are push-ups, freestyle squats and lunges, sit-ups, back stretch and chin ups. A good number is 10-20, even 30 of each.
→ Sports: Sports and Recreations are fantastic to have fun and excitement

while you are also, indirectly, getting health, fitness and exercise. Sports almost trick you into getting fit, where you would work up a sweat in no time.

→ Martial Arts: A boxing bag at Gym or home can help. Some jabs and kicks are great exercise to begin with. Learning the basics of self-defense is very helpful and should be used with caution and protection. You can think ahead and come up with your own style as self-defense classes tend to be a bit slow as they concentrate on 1-2 or 3 moves at a time. There are some good information and videos on YouTube and the Internet, DVDs and cable television.

However, be careful if aggression levels get bit high. My mate summed it up with – 'who on Earth are you going to fight, and what good would you do?' For example, Insight/Dateline on ABC or SBS had a show on youth violence and its devastating effects. It is suggested to use diplomacy and people skills first, then, if you must, self-defense. A wrestle is better than a punch and or kick as it as more passive and indirect, and shows you do not want to really hurt the person.

- *Therapy/Stress Management*
  → Sometimes, negative thoughts, feelings and actions, like stress, pain, tension and pressure, can be beneficial, in the right does and level. Being aware of this is better, beneficial and empowering, while not being aware of these negative things can be problematic. People would usually need some form of therapy and stress management to deal with these negative things.

  Natural Therapies (Meditation/Deep Breathing, Massage, Acupuncture). Private Health Insurance (E.g. BUPA/HCF) can cover this for free or at a discounted rate, with a number of visits offered throughout the year.

  Meditation/Deep Breathing (1-2 times a day – 20 minutes on a chair, lounge, bedroom or in backseat of car – refer to Mindfulness Meditation CD). My Dad survived 20 years of Bus Driving, whilst other drivers lasted 6 months or 1 year, with assistance of meditation/deep breathing. He learned this from an Indian Ushroom.

  My Dad combined this Meditation-Deep Breathing with strategies like a spiritual-religious following and a good meal at lunch time (My Dad a broken shift – morning and mid-afternoon).
  → Massage 1-2 times a week with either Massage Therapist or PainPod electronic device.
  → Acupuncture Relieves stress and pressure in points of the body that are affected.
  → Therapy/Stress Management supplements – Valerian, Passionflower, Cal-Mag (GNLD), Anti-Oxidants (Vitamins C, E, A and B), Zinc, Kava.
  → Alternative food/drink (consumed in balance; good to treat Lipoprotein Little A in blood): One-to-two times in the day, in a smaller glass - Coffee,

Wine/Whiskey, Cheeses, small rich portions of savory and sweet food.
→Herbal teas (Peppermint, Chamomile, Green tea, Lemon);
→ Shower (1-2 times a day; an extra shower can help you relax, and you can also do some meditation/deep breathing whilst in shower);
→ Hot or Cool Bath (once a week; provides another option to a shower and can do some meditation/deep breathing whilst in bath).
→ Warm Milk/Tea: Perhaps with some honey or ginger.
→ Spices mixture: Ginger, garlic, honey, lemon or lime, chilli, apple cider vinegar and turmeric. Good for a number of things, including a blocked heart, cold and flu and cleansing blood and arteries.
→ Garlic cloves Swallow or chew on 1-2 Garlic cloves each day, which is good as an antiseptic and cleanse.
→ Cold & Flu: Lemon & Honey, Eucalyptus Oil (can put on tissue or hanky, in boiling water, inhale it or under bed, inhale from steam machine), swallow and or chew on Garlic, Warm Milk/Tea, Vicks
→ Nasal Spray: One spray per nostril 1-2 times a day. Good for prevention and early detection. Many around like Rhinocort and Sudafed.
→ Dry-Eye Drops from chemist, e.g. Systane.
→ Comedies: Comedies are good for laughter and positivity, and if the show is good and funny enough, also some good exercise and healing like a hearty belly laugh. Make a list of comedy shows or movies and buy or hire them out, for example, Comedy Channel, YouTube, Soap Operas, Google Play, iTunes, Benny Hill, Mr. Bean, mainstream television.

- *Medication:*
According to top Australian Cardiologist and Health presenter, Dr. Ross Walker, if one lives in this modern era, with various factors affecting one's health, like stress, diseases and illnesses, pollutants and additives to food and various products, then sometimes medication is needed. Medication is so powerful nowadays that it can even keep you alive. One must be careful with certain medications as they can have side effects. The Internet is a great place to check up on a medication, and mention to a trusted health professional.

- *Medical*
→ Be careful of tests and diagnoses from doctors; they are stereotypically there to prescribe medication and do surgical procedures. Always get a second or third opinion, do some research on the Internet which has a wealth of information, try and use natural or alternative health and or remedies, for example, as mentioned under Health, and more importantly, see a spiritual advisor like a charismatic Priest or Pastor or Spiritual Advisor as they can have something significant to state to you about yourself and your life.
→ There is a battle between the medical field and alternative or natural remedies. Both think they are correct but really both have something to offer and should be working in with one another. If one had to be correct it would be the alternative or natural remedies first as healthy living and a healthy diet helps further in a prevention and early detection, for example, diet, exercise, therapy

and stress management and personal development, is better than any medicine.

But if a person already has a sickness, illness or disease, and has progressed ahead, then a combination of alternative-natural treatment with mainstream medicine can be beneficial.

→ Doctors have done autopsies on deceased patients, from heart disease, cancer, stroke and even suicide, and found a lot of, what Dr. Ross Walker (top Australian Cardiologist and Health Presenter) and American Dr. and Presenter, Russell Blaylock, 'bad chemicals'/ 'free radicals'. So the idea is to consistently deal with and flush out these bad chemicals/free radicals to live a healthier life and be free from various sicknesses, illnesses, diseases and stresses.

However, and this is true too, but some bacteria in the body is beneficial to combat these sicknesses, illnesses, diseases and stresses. A good example is poorer, second world and third world countries, where the people are around bacteria, and yet, survive and live to a long or relatively long age. So a blend of good food and health and some bacteria. There was a documentary on the importance of bacteria in the body on ABC/SBS television a while ago.

→ It is important to have a Blood test every 6 months to a year, full body test/examination, CT scanning of your arteries (See hand-out), Stress/Cardiology test for Heart and body (Dr. Ross Walker), Ultra-Sound of stomach organs and heart, MRI especially of Head and body, Gastroctomy/Endoscopy (for intestines and bowel).

→ <u>Private Health Insurance:</u>
The Australian Government is encouraging people to have Private Health Insurance, especially with the huge Medical-Medical Sickness debt. 'Health is Wealth', and people should not take any chances or risks with their health. The monthly Health Fund insurance bills cover you for a host of areas, like Dental, Optical/Vision, Natural Therapies (e.g. Massage, Acupuncture and Physiotherapy/Chiropractor) and Hospital (general and psychiatric). Some common and popular health insurers are HCF, BUPA/Medibank Private and NIB.

To highlight the power of Private Health Insurance, I was in a psychiatric hospital in Sydney, after being ill for a while. I paid a monthly payment of $170-$190, including psychiatric treatment. For the month and a half I was in this private hospital in Sydney, my BUPA health insurance covered for $25,000. This $25,000 is an absolute huge amount, and I was ever so grateful and lucky to have taken out this type of health insurance cover in time.

- *Other Factors (Mental/Psychological, Emotional, Physical and Spiritual/Religious)*

  A person might have previously or currently been affected by some problem, issue or sickness/illness that has created a block in their health and life. Finding trusted family or friends, a counselor/psychologist/kinesiologist and spiritual/religious advisor can help in finding out why it is taking a long time for you or somebody else to heal. Sometimes a block can be there for a reason and it is important to find this out, looking at all factors of life – Mental-Psychological, Physical, Emotional, Soul and Spirit and Spiritually and Religiously. The block or illness may be there as a form of cleansing and purgatory, as stated in the Christian teaching.

- *Personal Development*
  → Books, booklets, Journal Articles, Internet, CDs, DVDs
  → Write a 'Goals'/'Planning' list as to what you need and want in your life. There is a saying, 'Goals not Gifts, are more beneficial'. Just imagine how far you can reach, and what you can achieve in your life, with proper plans and goals if you have not used them until now.
  → Spiritual/Religious: Joyce Meyer, Joel Osteen, David Jeremiah and Father John Corapi (YouTube and Australian Christian Channel – ACC – on Cable and Catholic Television Network - CTN).
  → Relationships: Alan Pease CD, 'Relationships', and Alan Pease Book - Why Men Don't Listen and Why Women Can't Read Maps (see Sheet).
  → Health: Dr Ross Walker (top Australian Cardiologist and Health Presenter) Talk, 'Balance is Everything', given at Network 21 conference; Has book '5 stages of Health' (see print out) and has program on 2UE (see sheet).
  → Health: Dr. Russell Blaylock M.D. – 'Health and Nutrition Secrets' book and audio CD from Internet. Also had interview with Nutritionist Mike Adams, under Truth Publishing, on Internet.
  → Health: Deepak Chopra CD – 'Magical Mind, Magical Body (see Sheet)
  → People/Relationships: Skills with People, Les Giblin (see Sheet); Allan Pease, 'Relationships', from Network 21 audio CD.
  → Health/Spiritual-Religious - Grant Mullen: Pastor-Physician – Said how the most type of people who came to see him were Christians, how they concentrated on the soul-spirit, but not on other parts of the body (Mind, Body and Emotions). The opposite for people who concentrate on the body, but not on the soul-spirit.
  → General Personal Development: Paul Hanna, Book, 'You Can Do It' (see Sheet). A fantastic brief, all-round book. You may find another personal development publication similar to Paul Hanna's.

2. **Activities**
    - Goal: Some time for people in your life.
    - Goal: Work part-time, casual or volunteer in certain area to free up time to do the things that are important in your life.
    - Goal: Simplify life in general (simplicity in complexity and complexity in simplicity).
    - Goal: Help yourself, and your family and friends, be more financially sound to do the things they would like to do in their life.

General

- Some people can be too lazy, others too busy, and others up and down and too all over the place. The idea and point is to find 'balance' that is relevant to each person. Someone who is not dating, not going out or not married to somebody might cherish their work and activities and things in their life even more so. This might not mean they are missing certain things in their life, it is just they are content where they are and with what they are doing at the moment. That work, activity or thing might mean more to them than to somebody else. The person might find someone to go out with or marry, or do something when the time is right for them. However, it is always good for a person to find out by checking up on a person if they are alright as a person might be over- or under- working, or becoming sick or ill, or can still improve or develop a certain area or areas of their life if they choose to or allow it.

Work

- → Some people spend all or most of their life in a job/career, while others might go from job/career to job/career.
  → Are you comfortable and satisfied with where you are or do you need a new challenge?
  → Is there any tasks, roles and skills in your current job/career and business/company that you have not done or achieved?
  → Would you like to be an Executive, Manager, or maybe a few levels down as an Assistant Manager, Supervisor or Team Leader?
- Instead of doing another course, undertake some volunteer, work experience or work for lower pay. With this, you become like a free-wheeler and learn a number of things which you would probably not learn in a course or just one, long-term job/career/role. Or you would talk about it in the course (theory), but not do it (practice/work).This shows a true love for work/job/career and the skills and talents earned are priceless/golden and can turn into money, sooner or later.
- Another point is, some people love their job, and there is nothing wrong with that as 'life is a prayer'. Like above, this shows a true, honest, deep love for work. It is just the way one goes about it. Perhaps you might be obsessed and addicted to your job more than you should be, or stressed and sick from your job, or doing two or more jobs when there is no need to do all this work.

Life is too short to let life pass you by. American Christian Pastor-Presenter Joyce Meyer said how everyone these-days is in a hurry with no time to enjoy their house, children or life.

Education
- Education, combined with other fields, like Health and Fitness and Sport and Recreation, Work, Faith and Relationships, provides an important structure, organization and foundation for a person's life. With Education, together with the other fields/areas, people learn to address and deal with each type of stimulus, experience, learning and performing. The aim is to be constructive and aim for 'lifelong learning', or a 'student for life'.
- There are some good short courses and the like around – Private Industry Institutes, Community Colleges, TAFE, OTEN (study from home), Workers Education Association (WEA) and courses through Centrelink. University is good, but can tend to complicate an area with theory-too much theory for a practical field. Usually, in general, jobs/careers/roles in the workplace are more straightforward, with some of what was studied being incorporated now and again.
- Younger students should also be allowed to enjoy their education in the earlier years, like primary, and learn some things about themselves, for example how they learn (written, visual, auditory) and their personalities and characters.
- *Tutoring:* Tutoring should be used wisely for students, whether it be in the earlier and or later years of education. Some learn early in life, while others learn later in life, and some a combination of both. One should look at themselves, or through others, if tutoring, i.e. extra education, makes them relax their guard, and either become lazy or over-work/workaholics.
- Is there an area you would like to look at or research more? Perhaps your work might offer something or there is always the library, personal development material or the Internet.

Investment
- In today's society, we live in an era where 'wealth creation' is more prevalent compared to previous years. Jobs and money, and paying bills and debts, were easier to come by in previous years compared to today where things are harder. This means more people are looking for other ways to survive, earn money and make ends meet.
- These forms of making money are recommended for those who are not surviving with their current job/s and need some extra help or just to be comfortable, and for others, rich.
- From a spiritual viewpoint, God is a creator, so it is a blessing to be able to create something from time-to-time. I recommend some self-control with this.
  → Insurance: Example – 'Insurance Line' – For $20-30 a fortnight can cover you for $2000-$3000 for 3 months up to 24 months if need be for bills, unemployment, sickness or injury. Life Insurance is important in case of sickness, injury and death for the remaining family and to even pay off the

mortgage remaining on a house/apartment/building.

→ Product Creation Perhaps something creative or artistic, information-based, exercise or sporty, or just a very good idea for a product. Can look at the TVSN (Television Shopping Network), Danoz Direct or Penny Miller or Innovations magazines for the basis for your idea. I recommend best not go overboard with this; just one or a few good workable ideas are fine.

→ Information (work and non-work related, e.g. research, essays, reports, studies, stories/articles, booklet, on your own web-site). There is LinkedIn or you might create an e-book or make a hard-copy or make a small online or hard copy newsletter or newspaper. Again, best not go overboard with this in general.

→ Networking: Network21-Amway, Isagenix, GNLD and USANA.

→ Artistic Painting, drawing, sculpting, writing

→ Technical Trades and Hobbies and Interests, like Woodwork/Carpentry/Building, Metalwork, Electronics, Handyman.

→ Cultural Different elements of a nationality, culture and religion.

→ Food/Drink You may make 2-4 plates/trays of food for say $50-$100. You can get some help from family and friends to quicken the preparation of the food and drink.

→ Own Business/Consultancy: You can be self-employed, in a partnership or employing a number of employees for a specific or interested product and or service. You can even be the boss/CEO/owner/manager and delegate work to employees under you and gain a small percentage from the wages/salaries of each of your employees. You can work on a minimal or maximal level.

Hobbies and Interests

- It is amazing how some people do not have a hobby or interest, young or old, but especially those in older life or nearing or just after retirement. It is very important to keep the mind, body and spirit occupied, especially at the lower-lazier times and then the opposite with harder-tougher times. My father, as a Bus Driver, family man and individual saw many people, in his home country of Ireland, the Bus Driving and in general, go down the road from not having some proper hobby or interest.

- Here are some examples of Hobbies and Interests you might have:

→ Charity work: You can join or contribute to a charity to help others, in Sydney or elsewhere. You may provide money and or physical assistance. There are many charities in Australia and worldwide. You can provide great assistance personally as well as helping the other person.

→ Personal Development: There is plenty of material around for help, guidance, advice and interest. There are publications, like Paul Hanna's 'You Can Do It', the Internet and shows on television for things you like. The aim is to be constructive and aim for 'lifelong learning', or a 'student for life'.

→ Exercise: Even just a walk down the street and back can do wonders. You can join a gym, do fitness at home, play a sport, and watching sport on the

Internet and television or cable.

→Socialising: Mix with family, friends, acquaintances and colleagues every so often.

→Television: There are a variety of television shows, like reality shows, soap operas, documentaries and news programs around on Cable and mainstream television like ABC and SBS on Australian television.

→ Internet: There are some more intellectual and analytical programs on Internet, as well as music (iTunes and Google Play) and information (Google, Yahoo and Ninemsn).

→ Various things: Artistic, Cultural, Technical, Business and Culinary (food and drink)

3.   *Faith*

- *Goal*: Increase spiritual-religious life, including charity work.
- Whereever you are in your Faith, if you believe in another Faith, don't pray or practice much, don't believe in Jesus or have had a bad experience of God in your life, you can make peace with your worldly life and eternal life with Heaven/Paradise. Why, because according to Christianity, Heaven/Paradise it is a better, homely place to be.

- If bored, sick or have problems, increase Faith as a part of a key strategy. Faith is one of the reasons why my Dad made it this far with his job in Bus Driving and life in general, including his troublesome past in his home country of Ireland. It is too risky to be unprotected with regards to Faith. Some who say they don't believe in God still know God exists, and state and act like they don't believe in God, but really do acknowledge deep down, but maybe want some more blessings and graces. These people could have also had some negative experience/s with spirituality-religion. This relates to the parable of the 'Prodigal Son'.

How the Prodigal/troublesome son came back to the forgiving Father (metaphor for God), despite what he had done. It is like an everyday person walking out the door of their home, only to walk back in the door of their home, at the end of the day, regardless of what happened during the day. This is symbolic for people returning to their Heavenly home in the eternal life; God wants you, wholeheartedly, to come back home to Heaven/Paradise. There is a place for you if you allow it. You can still make it to Heaven without having to believe in God directly. God understands his love and mercy is far greater than ours.

Another story is the parable of 'The Good Samaritan'. The Good Samaritan is like God, and we the victim needing assistance. The Good Samaritan helped an unrelated man, a sick and or injured person. We did not know God, or paid him/her much attention, but God knew us.

- There are some very powerful <u>Christian/Humanitarian lines</u>. Repeating these lines throughout the day is the same as stating positive affirmations:

→ 'There are many roads that lead to Rome (Heaven/Paradise)';
→ 'There are many Mansions in the Father's (God's) House';
→ 'Amazing Grace': 'Through many dangers, toils and snares, I have already come'.
→ 'We are Travellers on this Earth/World on a journey home (Heaven/eternal life);
→ 'Seek yea first the Kingdom of God, and his righteousness, and all these things shall be granted unto you, Alleluia';
→ 'I know the thoughts I think toward you says the Lord, to have you prosper, to give you a hope and a future, and an expected end. Then you shall come to me and hearken unto me, and I shall hear you, because I give you rivers in the desert, and Jackals and Ostriches shall bow down to you'.
→ 'Ask anything in my name (Lord/God), and it shall be granted'.
→ 'Fear not for I' am with you, be not dismayed for I' am your God. I will strengthen, I will help you, I will uphold you with the right hand of my righteousness.'
→ 'Come to me all who are burdened and heavy laddened, and I will give you rest.'
→ 'The Lord is my shepherd; I shall not want. He maketh me to lie down in green pastures: He leadeth me beside the still waters. He restoreth my soul.'
→ 'I died [the Lord], so you all can live life to the full.'
→ 'I [the Lord God] will never forget you, my people.'
→ 'You [the Lord] are my refuge, my stronghold.'
→ 'I' am restless, oh Lord, until I'm in thy presence.'
→ 'One bread, One Body': 'Gentile or Jew, Servant or Free, no more. We are now children of God, not slaves.
→ 'Righteous Anger': Standing up for what is good and strong, right, just and merciful in our own lives and the lives of others. Similar to passage, 'Seek ye the first the Kingdom of God, and his righteousness, and all these things shall be granted unto you.'

- The following are some helpful steps and strategies for people in the the Catholic-Christian faith, other faiths, and people in general. You can do some or all of the following, depending on your situation and circumstances. Balance is the key:

→<u>Christian Pastors/Speakers</u>: Joyce Meyer, Joel Osteen, David Jeremiah and Father John Corapi (YouTube, Australian Christian Channel (ACC) and Catholic Television Network – CTN).
→<u>Place of Worship</u> (Church/Temple/Mosque/Centre/Room): Can visit Church for prayer and contemplation, worship, ask for help and support, for guidance and to give thanks. The Mass/Place of Worship is one of the highest forms of

prayer. There are different elements to the Mass/Place of Worship, with the Holy Sacraments, rituals and procedures, fellowship, talks and music, all working in together.

→Holy Sacraments (Mass) – Baptism, Eucharist/Communion and Confession/Reconciliation. Our Pastor Brother Terry Fernando strongly emphasizes these sacraments, combined with other areas of Faith, Health and Life, to help people with problems, and to attain a miracle.

→ Personal prayers and petitions (see attached sheet for 'One-Liners prayers and statements' – This is your personal conversation/dialogue with the Heavenly/Eternal realm. They can be one-liners, statements and sayings in between the mainstream spiritual/religious prayers of a person's Faith, like:

- I pray for everyone in the world, on Earth, and everyone in the eternal life. I pray for the lives in this world and that we can make the most of it, keeping in mind the big picture with our home in Heaven and our eternal home.

- I pray that people can pour into Heaven, from the world, the Earth, from the different realms and worlds in the next/eternal life, from Purgatory, and even those from Hell who have suffered enough.

- I pray that people can pour into Heaven in their millions and billions, having a constant flow, where there is endless room like the vast universe, with endless love, understanding, forgiveness and mercy.

- I pray for our mental-psychological, physical, emotional, soul-and-spirit, and spiritually and religiously.

- I pray for our 'Health', 'Activities', 'Faith' and 'Relationships'.

- I pray for our 'Health' (Diet, Exercise, Therapy and Stress Management, Personal Development and Image, Presentation and Personal Hygiene)

  I pray for our 'Activities' (Work, Education, Hobbies and Interests, Health and Fitness and Sport and Recreation, Faith and Relationships)

  I pray for our 'Faith' (Soul-and-Spirit, Spiritually and Religiously, our lives in this world and our lives in the eternal life.)

  I pray for our 'Relationships' (Families, Relatives, Loved Ones – Husbands and Wives, Boyfriend and Girlfriend – Friends, Acquaintances and Colleagues)

- I pray for, Goodness and Strength; Control and Constructiveness; Steadiness and Stability; Happiness and Content; Love and Understanding;

Wisdom and Knowledge; Patience; Trust; Care; Loyalty; Faithfulness; Peace, Calmness and Tranquillity; Humility-Humbleness and Strength; Diplomacy and People Skills; Conflict Resolution; Risk Management; Balance; Structure and Organisation; Planning and Goal-Setting; Self-Esteem; Motivation; Enthusiasm; Confidence; Determination; Perseverance and Persistence; Resilience; Forgiveness; Courage; Positivity over Negativity.

- I ask for these prayers in the name of Our Lord and Saviour and or Jesus Christ Our Lord; Our Lady, Immaculate Conception, Virgin Mother, Mother Mary; Holy Spirit, Holy Son; Holy Father; Angels (Guardian Angels and Arch Angels) and Saints and Celestial Beings.

- Then, 'Our Father', 'Hail Mary', 'Glory Be', 'Eternal Rest grant unto them Our Lord', 'Oh My Jesus/Lord...', 'Eternal Father I offer you...'/ 'I Believe, I adore, I hope, and I love thee...'

- Spiritual advisor: Someone from Church/Place of Worship, e.g. Priest, Pastor or Healer (in Society/Spiritually/Religiously), especially Charismatic, or someone you know who has a good spiritual-religious outlook on life, is good and strong and or willing, and can give you good advice, guidance and assistance. Examples are the 'Catholic Charismatic Renewal/CCR' and 'Divine Retreat Centre', Somersby, Gosford (who have come all the way from Kerala in South India).

Healing: Get someone well-controlled and strong to pray/lay hands over you frequently, or attend a healing group or mass, often, nearby to you, for example, from Church/Place of Worship or local community, CCR and Divine Retreat Centre or individual healers who visit from time-to-time. If there is nothing on offer in your Place of Worship, local area, or near to you, you should take the first steps to establishing a Healing group and or service.

To illustrate the power of 'laying hands', a lady was waiting in a Hospital waiting-room, in shocking pain, waiting to see one of the doctors. She remembered about prayer, and quietly said a prayerful statement. Out-of-the-blue, a male nurse went up to her, laid his hand on her head, said a few words under his breath, and then went away. The lady not only felt better, but she got up, left the Hospital waiting room, and went home.

If this sort of healing does not work, and only if it does not, you may have to visit someone or a group who is magical, divine or has supernatural powers, in the Church, from other Faiths and even Atheists. For example these sorts of people call themselves 'Healers-Sages'; they are like you and me but have progressed in their journey and experience of life and have a good blend of worldly and spiritual knowledge. It is recommended that you filter what they say because some wisdom and knowledge and power can be subjective and personal and exploratory, for example, taking certain drugs and medication, and relaxing of moral values and boundaries.

There are also others from other religions, such as a Monk from Buddhism, Imam from Muslim and Hindu Priest from Hinduism. An example of this is meditation, Yoga and Ayurvedic medicine and information. These religions have been around for centuries and would have picked up and learned some useful ideas, strategies, information and actions over those years. However, it is best to be careful with this and do your research before you go. Some practitioners get you to go through their rituals and procedures, but if you are smart, it is best to just pick the main thing or things that can help you and use them constructively as part of your short journey in this life.

- Being like Jesus: In Jesus time, the Disciples, James and John, were the closest to Jesus at the time. Both James and John would argue, who is like Jesus. Despite James and John having strengths, Jesus reminded them that he was the one who was carrying the burden, that Jesus was the Messiah. So when someone says, to be like Jesus, you do it in your own unique way, keeping balanced as best you can, with not too much, or too less.

- Spiritual and Religious information: This is to fill your mind constructively with good things, e.g. Holy Bible/text, study guides, literature, books, CDs, DVDs, Internet, pictures. You select, or another trustworthy person select, some good, strong and proper lines, statements and paragraphs to go over, like a prayerful positive affirmation, goal or plan. Just a bit each day can help. Study guides and Bible Study are good because interpreting the Holy Bible by yourself can mislead you, and it needs proper interpretation or to just confirm you are right.

A good example of a very influential booklet is, 'The Daily Journal', a Christian publication (see attachment copies), combining spiritual-religious information with everyday living.

- Charity/Helping people – When you help people a mega-endorphin enters your body called DiDorphin. My former boss and friend, who was also a Christian, stated this to me. When you show love for your fellow person, this comes back to you in some way or another. Aim to be sincere as best you can, or if not, keep persisting and the sincerity will eventually follow.

Try not to expect anything back in return from the people you help, as it will, surely, come back or be given to you someday, sooner or later, in this world and the eternal life.
- Advice to people: If you have some wisdom and knowledge and understanding on certain things, or referring them to someone else properly-equipped, share it with someone who needs it from time-to-time from the different areas of your life and people you meet and mix with. There's no need to go overboard but a

bit can help.

- <u>Giving your life/Taking the Blame</u>: There is no need for a Christian and non-Christian to give their life, like a martyr. The mechanics are there, and the hard-work has been done in the early years of Christianity and the early martyrs. Such an issue relates to giving the Lord/God your life and everything, in theory. The Devil/Evil-Bad spirit is cunning by tricking you into giving up your short precious life, for example, re-introducing martyrdom and the Defence forces such as the Army.

- <u>Spiritual-Religious things to take notice of in society</u>:
Music:

Bob Marley: 'One Love' – 'Is there a place for the hopeless sinners, who have hurt all mankind.' (Yes there is a place, in Heaven/Paradise, for these sinners and others)

John Lennon, The Beatles: 'Imagine' – 'Imagine there is no Heaven...' (Sorry John, imagine there is a Heaven/Paradise)

Guns 'n Roses: 'It's so easy (functioning of life/going to Heaven/Paradise)...'
'Knocking on Heaven's door'
'Take me now to the paradise city, where the grass is green and the girls are pretty'

The Script (Ireland – Danny O'Donohue): 'I'm still alive but I'm barely breathing. I pray to a God who I don't believe in'.

Daughtry (America – Chris Daughtry): 'It's not over' – 'It's not over. I'll try to make it right this time around. It's not over. Half of me is dead and in the ground. This love is killing me, but you are the only one.'

Live (American – Ed Kowalsick): 'I don't need no one to tell about Heaven. I look at my daughter, and I believe. I don't believe in proof, in God and truth. I can see the sunset and I believe

'...and the greatest of teachers won't hesitate, to leave you there by yourself chained to your fate

James Blunt (Englishman and former British Soldier): 'They came down from Heaven. Smoked 9(am) to 7(pm). All the stuff that they could find. Now they are really sorry for what they have done. They were just three wise men just trying to have some. (Again, do not take this literally. Done properly and moderately.)

4. ***Relationships***
    - Goal: More time for family and people in your life.
    - Goal: Keeping close to family and friends is important.

    - <u>The World is here for us:</u> Without people in this world, it would be worthless. The world, the Earth, has been put here for us. Compared to previous and or ancient years ago, most people lived to a big old age. However, life is shorter these days, for a number of reasons, so when will we have another human experience like this again. In stating this, it is best to tread carefully in life, keeping in mind the big picture, and live our worldly, human lives with our eternal lives in mind.

    - <u>Human/People/Diplomacy skills:</u> Previous generations did not know much about people relations and skills, like we do today, for example, controlling conflict, listening to someone and building up the hopes, dreams, needs and wants of a person/s. There is a plethora of people relations material and publications around to help us, for example, Les Giblin's 'Skills with People', Paul Hanna's 'You Can Do It' and Allan Pease's 'Relationships'. With modern life, publicly and privately, being stressful, people relations has never been more stretched and exhausted than ever before, for examples, bills and mortgages, two partners working, long hours, food quality, pollution (e.g. air and water), and shorter time span for relationships and marriages.

    - <u>Keeping close to family and friends is important</u>. If a person/s has a good and strong family, stay close to it. Or, even just some good friends, acquaintances and colleagues. Marriages and Relationships are collapsing under modern living. People should make the decision to concentrate on their family and friends to make it work, as best they can. This goes to goals/planning, and what you focus on, grows, improves and develops. It can even be said that we will see our family and friends in the next life, the eternal life, preferably in Heaven.

    - <u>Finding someone in your life/ Relationship issues:</u> A single person should first go through family and friends to find someone in their life, as a sure first bet, as they care and love you and have your best intentions in mind. Only if this does not work, then confront the society out there to look for someone, for example, walking up to someone or online dating (e.g. eHarmony, RSVP or Catholic Match). Again, keeping the relationship simple and straightforward allows you to focus on other important things in life. Our parents and grandparents era saw long relationships, unlike today. I guess the thing is what do you want out of the relationship. But if you want to stay with the person, you would do what you can, within consideration, to make it work.

- <u>Socialising</u> – Do you know yourself? If you socialize too much do you become distracted, less focused and or succumbing to peer pressure. Learn to minimize or increase socializing, with the right balance in mind, to concentrate on the things you really want to do or are important in your life. Sometimes, it is also socializing for that greater good of helping and being there for others, still keeping in mind yourself. For example, American Christian Pastor and Speaker, Joyce Meyer, always wondered why she was kept away from certain things in life. She ended up finding out she was being kept for the big picture and more important things in life, to protect herself from the evil that is in the world, and to pass the word and assistance to people she meets and comes across, like Charity.

- <u>Forgiveness and Mercy</u> People's relationships can sometimes or often call upon 'Forgiveness' and 'Mercy'. Gods love, understanding, forgiveness and mercy is well beyond us. He knows we are sinners, with most of us being good, and that we long for better lives, in this world and in Heaven and our eternal life.

My Father visited my Grandfather's brother, my Grand-Uncle, after so many years, following a fallout in the family many years back in Ireland. His Grand-Uncle even said nasty words and comments directly to my Dad in the past in Ireland, being a foul-mouthed drunkard, with a good heart and fantastic sense of humor, somewhere in there. My Dad gathered the courage, and buried the past, by visiting his Grand-Uncle, who happened to live in the Sydney area. You would not believe it, but it turned my Grand-Uncle's life around; he was so happy. He later died soon after, but he was so happy to have been forgiven and to have made better relations among the family. Paul Hanna, mentions this in his book, 'You Can Do It', on the chapter on 'Forgiveness'.

- <u>Organisations</u> – Local community health centres, Relationships Australia NSW, Family Planning NSW and The Australian Family Association

- <u>Societal/Worldly issues:</u>
- *Food and Drink and Health*
- *Drugs and Substance Abuse*
- *Length of modern relationships and marriages/Growth of de facto-partnerships*
- *Gay and Lesbian relationships*
- *Multi-Skilling privately and publicly*
- *Women in the workforce*
- *Stress and Time Management*
- *Gambling*
- *Violence and Sex (publicly and privately)*

Health: What's up Doc?
Talk about the health and medical system in Australia

'Health is Wealth', as the saying goes, but this seems to be lost in an Australian health and medical system that doesn't look like it is going to be fixed anytime soon.

Where do you start with a system as this at the moment? There is a current health and fitness boom, in what is a fast-paced, stressful and technological society, but the end result is like a see-saw going up and down. Some become are healthy whilst others are not. Some are becoming sick whilst others are not. It is almost like the gap between rich and poor. It is true it takes all kinds to make a world, and people are different and will do different things compared to one another, and this also applies to the health and medical system.

One thing is for sure, we are very lucky, and should be thankful to be living in the modern era. Our parents and grandparents never knew or experienced what we have today - weight control, anti-ageing, pregnancies, beauty and sexual health. The list goes on. There is a wealth of information on health and medicine on the Internet, libraries and health and medical departments, groups and organisations. Yet things still happen.

My father, being brought up in a traditional environment, said we as a people in the global village, have lost our moral values and become selfish and greedy. We have it all, we want it all, and yet problems keep rearing their ugly head. In the European countries of France and England there is both free health care and education. Now, Australia is a colonial country, in fact a democratic, first world country, but such a system as that which is in France and England has benefits and disadvantages. Free is good, everyone working towards or being healthy, but then some relax off and take it for granted. Then again, there is no harm in some help and leeway.

Revered and experienced Cardiologist, speaker and media personality, Dr. Ross Walker explained how you would have a supposedly healthy adult male or female, doing their exercise, eating healthy and getting some therapy and stress management, and are told by their local doctor/GP that their bad cholesterol is a bit high but nothing to worry about, and in a year or so they are dead.

Self-education is paramount these days and it is very important to come to the table, i.e. your local GP, with some knowledge and research to know what to test and look out for. But tread carefully. Imagine waiting 8-10 hours to see a doctor at your local or nearby hospital; first the local GP, then the local hospital. Some people have been terribly sick or in shocking pain waiting to see a doctor. Those in the know have to literally make tried and true song and dance to even get a look in at a respectful time. I personally know of a best mate whose sister died in the waiting room at his local hospital and my brother's best friend who made that song and dance, and if he didn't, his daughter could have died, being in a bad way.

I must say, the Rudd Government's 'Super Clinics' sounded like a very good idea to relieve the current hospital system. The problem is not getting to an operating table to begin with. Prevention and early detection are the key words here, but have become like fashion statements in the health and medical industry.

A very important element of prevention and early detection is spirituality; how life is a prayer. Some people overlook the spiritual realm for keeping healthy and or getting better from a sickness or illness. Prayers, a place of worship and a charismatic Priest or Pastor or someone in the spirit can help a person considerably. It would be a tremendous step to hear, for once, someone from the medical or spiritual side say, 'What can I do for you?' or, 'What element of your life do you need help with?'

My father lasted over 20 years in government bus driving, one of the toughest jobs in the world. My dad was never made for it, choosing to read a good book at the drop of a hat; yet he lasted that long, and one of the reasons was his faith and spirituality, also including some healthy eating and useful meditation. There are others like this as well out there I'm sure.

Then again there is such a thing in spirituality as a cross to bear, or the struggle of life. Perhaps this is what the Australian health and medical system is on about, your cross and struggle in life. Local Australian Personal Development speaker, Paul Hanna, mentioned if people knew how close they were to a better life or to a goal if they just persisted and did not give up. But as I stated earlier, there is no harm in a bit, or a lot...lots is good...of help.

Bibliography

- Personal experiences:
  - I thought about being a Life Coach at one stage, but decided to make my own areas of life that needed to be concentrated on, including Health (Also Activities, Faith and Relationships).

  - I personally being 'in the spirit', with my blend of worldly and spiritual knowledge having progressed so far.

Activities in Life

With the fact we have been put here on this planet to live our lives, we would have to do something in living these lives; we have to pass our time doing some Activities. Hence who knows when we will have such a free human experience as this? Activities can be work/job, education, hobbies and interests, socialising, sport and leisure, wealth creation and investments, etc.

1. Activities as Constructive

Some people think the world has become a wicked and greedy place, and it is true to some extent. There is also the Christian statement, '...you will work by the sweat of your brow', meaning life is a struggle. There is also the saying, 'An idle mind is a Devil's workshop'. This can also go the other way for people who are too busy, hence a balance is needed.
However, the essence of our community, society and worldly systems is beneficial and constructive. Just to live your life and experience such a life in an enjoyable and fulfilling way, taking in the struggle of life, is what it is all about.

2. Having Big Picture in mind

In undertaking these Activities, it is important to have the big picture in mind, i.e. Heaven and your Eternal Realm. There is a Christian song with words, 'seek ye first the Kingdom, and all these things shall be granted on to you'. Another saying is, **'you do the work** (i.e. Activities) **and stay away from the glory'** (the behind-the-scenes of the world and life like Supernatural and Divine, as this is God's realm). Although there are some people in society who partake in this realm, largely it is not to be touched.

In this way, life is a prayer. God is a creator and we have been blessed with different talents and skills, which we have learnt from birth, to make a good blend of worldly and spiritual knowledge and wisdom, for most people. So Jesus knows our need, want and desires to have these Activities in our lives. One would expect to have these Activities in Heaven and good parts of Hell too at certain times providing an extension of the worldly Activities on Earth.

3. Keeping it simple

Some people are so busy or lazy or all over the place they lack a balance for other things in life. Some people might want to keep it simple. For others, keeping it simple might mean being busy and or complex but in a proper and constructive way.
People lack that time for themselves and others, for example, considering working less hours, getting a part-time or casual job, looking after your health, a hobby or interest, sport and exercise, socialising and family and friends, a faith and charity. We don't get too many opportunities at life so we try and fit everything in. In the process, we forget about ourselves and or others and even our faith, depending

on what faith we follow.

It is time we looked at what is really important in our lives and concentrate on that, and 'keeping it simple' might be the way to go.

4. Activities help avoid Distraction

One has to consider oneself lucky because by keeping on track with the various Activities one does, keeps them out of trouble or distraction. The media is filled with story-after-story of so many incidents of people losing focus of life with bad things happening, for example, crime and violence. Would you want to be there or over here? As the saying goes, 'it is a wicked world but we don't have to be a part of it' or 'an idle mind is the Devil's workshop'.

5. Stressful, Fast-Paced World

Use of work, or a job, can be beneficial, but one has to look at the context it is coming from. Today, we live in a stressful, fast-paced society that can take the mere life from you if you are not careful. Some people are working two-to-three jobs to survive and or be comfortable. Some can handle this for a while, whilst others are walking a dangerous tight rope putting their lives at risk. From a Christian viewpoint, the Devil can sometimes use a job, let alone other things, to get you caught up in the world and or yourself. Have you heard of that saying, 'I'm sorry, I'm just too busy'.

Again you have to see where the person is coming from and if they have the big picture in mind. A person might be on their own, working, with no family, or working two-to-three jobs, but they are enjoying the hard work, and quite frankly it is their business. However it is always important to check on the person from time-to-time to see how they are going, especially in this day-in-age with things happening.

With the high cost of living the way it is, money has become a central issue in peoples' lives and society. Sometimes a job is not enough to make ends meet, and some people can go from job-to-job with the lifespan of a particular job being one-to-two years. In stating this, if a person is not making enough money or for some reason cannot get a second or third job, how will they make ends meet? This is a very powerful question because some people do not know anything else other than a job. Welfare through the Australian Government in Centrelink only offers so much. Enter the 'era of wealth creation'.

6. Era of Wealth Creation

There are a flood of ideas on how to make money, if one really needs it. However, nothing can beat an honest job to earn money and make ends meet as money can lead to greed and corruption.

Common ways to make money are Shares and Property/Real Estate but it is also good to have some other ways to make some money in these hard times. What I would recommend is obtain personal development material on wealth creation and educate yourself. Some examples are Networking or Multi-Level Marketing, creating a product or service (e.g. shopping channel or Danoz), being artistic or creative, offering food and beverages (non-alcoholic drinks preferably), information like producing a publication or blog or a business or small business initiative or project on the side.

Again the big picture is important here and not getting too greedy for money by being constructive. For example, some Relationships have broken up because of money and the lack of time, and quality time, given to the Relationship. There is also the Christian parable of the rich man, for example, the poor man Lazarus and the rich man.

Bibliography
- Personal experiences:
  - I thought about being a Life Coach at one stage, but decided to make my own areas of life that needed to be concentrated on, including Activities (Also Health, Faith and Relationships).

  - I'm somewhat 'in the spirit', with my blend of worldly and spiritual knowledge having progressed so far.

Relationships these days

It is true people are the most important thing in existence. The world would not exist if it was not for people. God made the world for us people.

1. Human life a Gift from God

In stating this, people were put here to live their lives, as human beings, as human life is a gift from God. Hence the statement, 'we are pilgrims in this life, on a journey home'. However it is the way one lives their life that is the key and difference.

We have people in various areas of our lives, from family and relatives and loved ones like boyfriends and girlfriends and husbands and wives to friends, acquaintances and colleagues. There are people in our inner circle and those outside our inner circle.

Some people like being on their own, but would need a person or people from time-to-time, as it is hard to do it on your own these days.

2. Live a Better Life

Make the decision to live a better life, in a bit, some or all parts of your life. It is about finding your balance in life and being comfortable relevant to yourself. Yes there is struggle, or you may be lucky and have lived a perfect life, but taking in all the areas of the Life Plan – Health, Activities, Faith and Relationships – one can make it through in this life and the eternal life. This means deciding to be good and strong as best you can, keeping in mind being strong to protect and further your goodness to yourself, others and Heavenly and eternal life.

3. Human Relations has progressed

People have progressed a great deal from previous years when we did not know much about how people functioned. There is information on people skills and health and the mind and body more than ever before. What this has created is two groups, one who understands and functions properly and the second group who does not understand it and is not operating properly.

The Australian Government have even created an organisation called 'Relationships Australia'. Whether it is good or not is worth investigating, but the intention and idea is there.

4. Lack of Spirituality and Balance Today

Despite all this information and advancement, there seems to be a gap, something missing. Some might say, that is how it is, others might say it is the lack of spirituality and a balanced approach to life. Our parents and grandparents era did not know as much as we know now, yet they made their relationships last. Perhaps simplicity is best, as the saying goes, 'keep it simple stupid'. Then again, there is simplicity in complexity and complexity in simplicity. Additionally, another problem is not having enough time for the people in one's life. Pastor and renowned speaker, Joyce Meyer, stated how people are too much in a hurry to enjoy their house, their children and their life in general; again, this comes down to balance.

5. Relationships under Attack

Relationships are under attack, more so nowadays than in previous years, with divorce rates too high, people having too many sexual partners and getting sexually transmitted diseases, the growth of de facto relationships, both partners working as opposed to the wife or girlfriend staying at home, domestic violence, racism and multiculturalism and the spike in gay and lesbian relationships which never existed in previous generations.

From a spiritual and religious viewpoint, the Devil, or evil, is on the attack against relationships. A number of things come to mind here. Firstly, a family, or a couple, who prays together stays together. Let's just make it simple and say a family who stays together. Secondly, a balanced life is important with mental and psychological, physical and emotional and personal and personal, spiritual and religious. So the question remains what area of a person's life needs altering and fixing.

Bibliography

- Personal experiences:
  - I thought about being a Life Coach at one stage, but decided to make my own areas of life that needed to be concentrated on, including Relationships (Also Health, Activities and Faith).

  I personally being 'in the spirit', with my blend of worldly and spiritual knowledge having progressed so far.

Faith

This is the most important part of the Life Plan because it deals with the big picture of our lives on this Earth and our Eternal lives. If you were to die today, where do you think you would be going in your Eternal life, Heaven or Hell?

Faith can be, and is for most, a very significant part of a person's life, whether it is directly through religion or as a good living Atheist. A Christian Pastor once said Faith goes together with Hope and Love. So Faith on its own needs other elements.

Faith can be 'personal, spiritual and religious'. Usually it is a combination of the three. 'Personal' is how we treat ourselves and others and is our conversation with the Eternal Realm and God. 'Spiritual' is how we go about our daily lives and how 'life is a prayer' and has different degrees of spirituality, either directly or indirectly, for example, directly through meditation and exercises like Yoga or indirectly through one's daily Activities (refer to Activities).

'Religion' can be a sensitive issue for some yet it provides an important foundation for one's worldly and spiritual life. Going through the different rituals and procedures of one's religion is like positive affirmations and creates routine and structure to one's like. Even wonders and miracles can be performed through Religion that can leave people in society and the world baffled and amazed, for example, those in science and medicine. One cannot deny the existence of a presence in the world that keeps things together and functioning. Some call it God, others similar things.

There are a number of subjects to be discussed in relation to Faith:

1. Different religions and cultures.
2. Societal and Spiritual Figures
3. Joining the Spiritual-Religious roles/positions
4. Atheists
5. Supernatural and Divine Presence
6. Seeing family and friends in Heaven/Activities in Heaven
7. Jesus as being constructive
8. You do your best and God does the rest
9. Sin
10. Heaven, a better place and End-of-world talk
11. Rituals and procedures in a religion
12. Literature in a religion

1. *Different religions and cultures*

As the saying goes, 'we are one, but we are many'. This applies to different religions and cultures in our world. There is the microcosm, us as belonging to a certain religion and culture and society, and the macrocosm, of us being human beings.

One has to understand we are not like the animals that do not have much of a brain and conscience like human beings. Yet some people act as if they are animals in today's world.

Another saying is that 'there is good and bad in every race'. Whether you are rich or poor, strong or weak, good-looking or not good-looking, dress nicely or do not dress nicely, everyone deserves to be in a Faith on a spiritual and religious level. **Through God, have mercy on one another as God would have mercy on us, showing acceptance and tolerance for each other.** To support this, there is a Catholic-Christian hymn, 'One Bread, One Body', which states the words, 'Gentile or Jew, servant or free...'. In other words, we all can be worthy of Jesus and Heaven if we allow it.

There are the religions of Christianity, Buddhism, Islam, Hinduism, Black Magic and Atheism. There are Christian sayings, 'there are many roads that lead to Rome' and 'there are many mansions in the Father's house'. What this is saying is that we are different and we will take different paths in life. But there is a final destination, a better place to be, if people allow it. Some call it Heaven, others Paradise. Yet when properly questioned, there is a sense of doubt and hesitation if the person really wants to go to Heaven or should be there.

There is another Christian statement, 'we are pilgrims in this life on a journey home', and guess where home is, you guessed right, Heaven, or that better place. What a powerful statement, and some who have no religion, do not practice their religion or have been left ignorant, would not be aware of such information. Whether you believe in Jesus or God or not, if you are from other religions, it is about coming back to your rightful home in Heaven, or a better place to be. Life is like a contract, with fine-print, and one should know this fine-print in order to reach Heaven, or that better place.

When one really gets to the point, there is a Heaven and Hell with Purgatory there as well. So there are some good and bad points of life and different cultures and religions, but we can say, we have lived our lives the best way we know how, we repent and say sorry, possibly some cleansing and we go home, to Heaven, or that better place. No need for judgement as this will happen on an individual basis as God wants us to come back to him.

One can say we should, if not have to believe in Jesus to reach Heaven, this better place to be. But what about people from other cultures and religions who do not, or are not accustomed to believing in Jesus. I can say now you are not going to change them and they will go to their graves with their beliefs, practices and values. Some flexibility and love and understanding should be shown here and Jesus should be offered to these cultures and religions as a source of help and assistance and guidance; that is if the person/s has some strategies to get through this life on Earth and through their eternal lives. These people might just need Jesus at some time.

2. *Societal and Spiritual Figures*

There are societal/worldly and spiritual figures and people amongst us with certain wisdom, knowledge and information that can be good and bad, positive and negative for us.

With the *'Societal Figure'*, usually we everyday people have a good or developing blend of worldly and spiritual and religious knowledge, wisdom and power. Those who are particularly good or make themselves known can sometimes be called 'Healers' or 'in the spirit' and 'Sages' (people with wisdom, knowledge and information).

These people have positives and negatives because positively, sometimes these people know more than the societal and spiritual figures, but negatively because some of the information they provide needs to be filtered as it is subjective and personal.

There are also people in the world, Societal and or Spiritual and Religious, who give the wrong impression about the world and God, and one must be aware of this. It is true God is more knowing and powerful than us and that power, through certain societal and spiritual figures, can be shown and experienced incorrectly.

It can even be the people close to us who can do it, for example parents, teachers, bosses and managers at work, politicians and the media. All these people can at times lead us down the wrong path, but at least the attempt is to be proper role models, and this often can occur. It is true, no one is perfect, and from the Christian perspective, we are sinners. But, despite being sinners themselves, it is the good and strong amongst us who must rule over the bad otherwise there would, at some stage, or eventually, be chaos. An example of this is a Priest or Pastor in Church who is deemed to be Holy to lead the congregation of parishioners and mass.

Sometimes our own father and mother at home can be Societal Figures, but if he or she is a proper role model. The societal figures out there have some knowledge and wisdom, but might also have some bad elements, habits or vices, such as smoking, drinking or drugs, sex and violence. These poor, weak or negative elements can detract the example this figure, and other figures give and again one must be aware of this.

For example, in Mullewa Prison in Silverwater, Sydney, there are three generations of family in the prison, each following one another and ending up in the same predicament. If one was to rely on nature, it would be hit-and-miss, so such people, even everyday people with problems, issues and vices and addictions, need help changing certain elements or their whole character; so help is sometimes, if not usually, needed on a private and or public level.

Some people do not know the connotations looking up to these Societal Figures. Usually such figures come with expectations that can involve responsibility yet also danger. It is the physical side that can be dangerous, for example, being brought into the supernatural or violence. Offering knowledge, wisdom and power is a positive thing of what these figures can offer. Some people in society usually use these societal figures, especially some bad ones, as examples for their own agenda. These people tend to be Devil-like, weak, negative or ignorant. There system is used, and sometimes, and even usually, has never been questioned or brought into analysis.

It is usually these individuals, as well as those who are not religious or do not practice a religion, who push unaware people into joining a higher role in a religion or spirituality, such as becoming a Priest or Pastor with the person becoming the religious figure sometimes lacking a proper, deeper, whole and heartfelt knowledge and understanding of what they are doing; they just believe the figure in question. Please be aware of this.

These figures behind this may sometimes do not want to hear spiritual or religious information from people and are usually unprepared to take in such information. They do not know the person who is spiritual and or religious is actually being equipped to deal with their Faith and life in general, or is aiming to pass on some proper wisdom and knowledge, which can be undertaken incorrectly or poorly. An example is being called a 'Preacher' for attempting to be spiritual and or religious.

This is where spirituality and religion come in because on your own, unprepared individuals come across these societal people and figures and have negative experiences. It is sometimes being traditional with the thinking of previous generations, who did not know or have what we have today, for example, People Skills and Personal Development, Internet and Counsellors and Pastors. An example is following in your father's or parents' footsteps with a profession or job and having poor lifestyle choices such as a diet and exercise. There is also the modern thinking of relaxed moral values and a fast-paced of life. Although this has been how life is for some people, it has been said to cause some negative circumstances.

Then there is the *'Spiritual Figure'*, such as a Priest in Christianity, Hinduism or

Buddhism, a Pastor in Christianity, or an Imam or Sheikh in Islam. Healers and Sages would indirectly come under this heading.

Although meaning well, a lot of these spiritual figures have been trained a certain way or along a certain path, and sometimes have been educated not to provide a solution to someone's problem, just like doctors and counsellors and psychiatrists in the medical field. A Catholic Priest might be charismatic ('in the spirit') whilst another Catholic Priest may not be.

However, a Spiritual Figure usually has something significant to say to a person. If they are truly 'in the spirit', they can look right into a person and see all the different problems and good points of your life. Some people do not have a prayer life or believe in God, and this amongst other things like Health, Work and Education and Hobbies and Interests and Relationships, can be the reason for things going wrong in their life and others in their life. Hence a balanced approach to life should be taken.

3. Joining the Spiritual-Religious roles/positions

It can be said that there will be individuals who will join a religious order as a Priest/Pastor, Guru or Sheik/Imam for example, Catholicism and Christianity, Islam, Hinduism, Buddhism and Atheism. Some people are meant for being part of these religious roles, others not, and some have potential. To join and be a part of a religious order takes a certain and training, and can be difficult in modern times with all the challenges/obstacles, problems, issues and temptations around. We need to pray for these members of religious roles, to have them be true, strong and meaningful to such a position. We have to acknowledge that they are Human like the rest of us, and can make mistakes.

However, some people in such religious roles, and those who are not but aware of how these roles function, are not fully aware of what is involved with the role. Some big problems with these religious roles are misguiding their congregation by what they say and act, violence, sexual abuse and offensive language. Religious roles in the modern era therefore need to be looked at and analysed.

Certain things need to be done for people in such religious positions. With what is going on in the modern world, a watering or simplification needs to be happen for religious roles. Some ideas is dividing the role of say a Priest/Pastor to lessen the burden and delegate the role to others, thereby strengthening the role/s, especially with a greater spread of wisdom and knowledge being passed around. These people can help and guide members of their congregation, lay hands and heal them and carry out the various activities of the once singular position.

For example, a Priest/Pastor may become an acolyte, deacon or elder, where they can have a wife or husband/boyfriend and girlfriend. Celibacy can tend to be one of the toughest characteristics for those in religious positions. It is so easy for members of the congregation or general public, to accuse or blame the person in the religious role for sexual and other things. An instance of this is the current situation between Cardinal George Pell of the Catholic Church, and a number of sexual-violence abuse victims over time. This is why, delegating or simplifying these religious roles can lessen the effects of these important positions, in case something goes wrong.

What we are seeing is a revolution, and evolution, in religious orders around the world, where members of religious roles need some assistance. As mentioned, allowing a person/group in a religious role/s to be married or de facto and possibly have a family, and delegating and training and educating the role/s to other members of the congregation. There are questions that need to be answered, for example, can I employ other areas of life, public and private, and society, into these religious roles. Also, does the person/s in this religious role/s carry it on into their next-eternal life, or does it remain only a once-off Earthly activity and experience.

4. Atheists

We tend to live in a modern world where there are relaxed moral values and practices, and this can be seen with the rise in Atheism, or no belief or faith in a higher or Supreme Being. With Atheism, moral values become relaxed when Atheists lead into or live destructive lives.

There is a saying, 'there is good and bad in every race', as the saying goes, and this includes Atheists. Some Atheists do not know any better and are ignorant of Faith to some or a full extent. Some Atheists have encountered a bad experience of God or have not had God taught to them in their upbringing. Some of these Atheists go on to live destructive lives. Others respect the moral order, despite not practicing any Faith, and live constructive lives, such as Atheist and author Richard Dawkins.

Even though an Atheist does not believe in God, they still have a chance to make it to Heaven, if they allow it, for example, by repenting/confession (Christianity) and attempting to live a good life.

From a Christian viewpoint, Jesus Christ not only came for good and righteous, but also for the sinners, which would include most of us, and this would include Atheists. It is true, evil has entered society and the Church these days, and some Atheists can be treated badly or sinners have taken over and have not been kept under control and the good and strong have been stopped from making decisions for the good of everyone.

Some Atheists in particular, and people in general, have been dragged or tempted into immoral, evil or weak behaviour, for example, drinking and smoking, and they know or do not know that their bodily and spiritual defences have been weakened and or have evil spirit/s in them. It is good to observe the person for a while, but if their bad behaviour persists, it is important to make lifestyle changes or see a trustworthy spiritual advisor for advice and guidance.

However, some Atheists can get to Heaven before other people because they have faced and encountered life full on, despite the risk of doing this. They have experienced and learnt a number of things along the way and may even be closer to Heaven than one thinks. This also applies to most Atheists who have been constructive as best as possible with their lives and some who have turned away from being destructive.

One thing that Atheists can teach people in a religion is that sometimes religion can be a bit too constrictive. Most people do not understand the mechanics of a religion, for example, can I do this, can I do that, and also showing proper love and understanding. It can be a bit too much and people put up with it and remain dissatisfied or leave altogether. The correct answer is that a good blend of worldly and spiritual knowledge needs to be there, a balance. One has to remember we are not in our Heavenly realm yet, so as human beings we will have a state of imperfection until we do so, hence another Catholic-Christian saying, 'My heart is restless O' Lord until we are in thy presence'.

5. Supernatural and Divine Presence

God is Divine. The word magical can be a sensitive word for some people, for example, evil connotations of a witch or wizard. But such magic is usually, especially these days, in the hands of God, the Supreme Being, as well as those who can, or attempt to control it like 'Healers' and 'Sages' in everyday society and spiritual and religious figures.

How the universe and the world came into existence is a miracle in itself. This kind of magical and divine power exists today in the world and eternal realm, not just through religion, but society in general, for example, Health, Science and Medicine for instance.

There have been healings and miracles in religion and elsewhere that society cannot explain. Some people in society are unaware of these healings and miracles, but may have strategies in place that can see them survive. One has to understand that members of Christianity and other religions sometimes have to keep searching for that Supernatural and Divine power, especially with evil entering religion, and have to educate and research themselves to get proper and sufficient help and assistance and guidance.

As stated before, although science and medicine has progressed so far, a spiritual advisor or figure can have something important to say to you or assist you in your healing or recovery. Prayer, one's place of worship and spiritual and religious figures and people with healing and deliverance abilities are also significant parts of one's spiritual and religious life and can provide Supernatural and Divine assistance. Living a healthy and balanced life and lifestyle in general, at minimum, can also assist this Supernatural and Divine healing.

There are also people in society, like you and me, who are 'in the spirit' or 'healers'. They have a blend of worldly and spiritual knowledge that can be beneficial and have had contact with Supernatural or Divine elements of life. It is best to find one of these persons from a Faith instead to make sure some good, strong protection is there and one is not mislead. An example is from myself where some people I was working with blurted out, 'he should have become a Priest', just happening to recognize I was under stress. It was then that three separate people came up to me and said the same thing happened to them but something told them inside it was incorrect; one in particular said, 'he (the Devil) doesn't have you yet'. That last statement changed my life about a lot of things, including my spiritual and religious life and taught me to be more careful and aware.

Now, possibly, at some time, in a controlled and secure way, one might have to turn to other faiths for help. Now for Catholics and Christians, I know what you are saying, how can this be when Jesus is 'the truth, the way and the life'; in other words, all the help and assistance and guidance should be there in the Church and those who come to the Church. To give an example, a Christian Physician-Pastor Grant Mullen stated how more Christians than anyone else came into his doctor's surgery. They had been to the Communion/Eucharist and Repentance/Confession, but still had problems in their life. Sometimes it was life and lifestyle changes, but also being aware of the spiritual realm and its influences. Two people I encountered stated that it was only when they got Baptised and became a Christian that they gave up their disrupting vices and addictions.

A person from a Faith may not have found proper help in time, so another Faith, like Buddhism, Islam or Hinduism can assist a person. The aim though is to be focused and strategic in what one is looking for. A person/s does not need to convert or really undertake the rituals and practices of the particular Faith. Usually the main problem is health and wellbeing, for example problems and issues with sickness and strength, possibly even being possessed by some evil spirits and getting them early on. This person looking for the help needs to focus on and search for the solution in a safe and proper manner.

There is also some form of 'Physicality' on Earth and eternal realm (Heaven, Purgatory and Hell). Most of the time people are in their Heavenly in a state of supreme peace, safety and happiness motionless in the spirit, or going through some cleansing and purifying and suffering in their eternal bodies in Purgatory and Hell.

In Heaven, there will be spiritual assistance in helping people be safe, happy and strong.

Use of storages/memory from previous supernatural situations involving divine spirit and essence will be used to assist, inform and strengthen human beings in the eternal realm in general.
In Heaven, Jesus Christ, God and Trinity and relevant Angels and Celestial Beings

will help keep Heaven safe and secure to have their fill for themselves and for everyone else.

Properly used Supernatural/Divine elements will be used to help, assist and provide for people in Heaven and Hell.

6. Seeing family and friends in Heaven/Activities in Heaven

Failing to plan is planning to fail and this includes our eternal life in Heaven, where we spend most of our time.

We must get in our minds that we will see our family and friends again in Heaven, if not eternal realm. And why not, as these are important members of our family and friends, who we spent much time with on Earth. This point works in together with the fact there are Activities in Heaven to keep us occupied and content.

The Trinity (Jesus, God and Holy Spirit), the Celestial Beings, Angels (General, Guardian and Arch Angels) and relevant Saints will help keep Heaven safe and secure so they can have their own fill and fill for everyone else.

7. *Jesus as being Constructive*

This is a very important subject because the name and figure of Jesus Christ can be misunderstood.

Jesus represented how to be a better human being, despite being a spiritual figure. His aim was to be constructive, provide help and assistance to people and give a positive example to the people of his time and throughout time until today.

For example, Jesus Christ was one man who conquered the almighty Roman Empire. Jesus existed during the time of the Roman Empire, and his teaching, especially the efforts of his Apostles, spread Christianity in such a way as to have such a profound effect on the World and Eternal life. In stating this, having the Holy Trinity in us is to have the Trinity work together with each other in harmony, for our own benefit. Some people and figures in society, going back to the section on *'Societal and Spiritual Figures'*, abuse the trinity to suit their own purposes, mistreating some people they have contact with.

Jesus Christ was also practical. Christianity is more than just reading the Bible, or a Holy book in a certain religion, and not doing anything with it. It is physically getting up and doing something with it, for example, charity work, donations, providing help and assistance and advice to people in need and earning an income for your family through your hard efforts at work. In stating this, there needs to be a balance in life. Some people are more complex and do more things or are deeper, whilst other people are more simple and straightforward, some people can mistake this for being lazy.

Jesus was said to be the correct path to Heaven, as in his words, 'I'm the way, the truth and the life.' This is a very powerful statement, which again can be misused and abused by certain societal and spiritual and religious figures. However, for people from other faiths, they can either use Jesus for assistance in reaching Heaven or a better place or just to know his help and guidance is there for them if they need or want it.

A Priest once said, 'Did the Father intervene when his Prodigal son went down the wrong road?' The Priest said this confidently. But something stirred in me, the Holy Spirit did its work, and said, 'But Jesus intervened. In fact, the New Testament is about a man named Jesus who intervened in helping others. Sometimes the case of the Prodigal Son is relevant, but sometimes, in fact most times, it is not needed; in other words, something should be done. The lesson here is we do not have to go to the extent of Jesus, but help out here and there with our own family and friends and those we come in contact with when need be.

In Australia, there are Churches everywhere, not for a joke, for a reason. If Christianity did not work as a religion, the decision-makers in our society would not have allowed such Churches to have been made.

8. You do your best and God does the rest

Some people think they can make it in life without Christianity or a religion or without being spiritual. These people may last for a while, even into older ages, but when problems or sickness hits, it can hit hard. By having Faith in your life, and a good balance in one's life, these problems and sicknesses can be overcome sooner or eventually.

There is a saying, 'you do your best and God does the rest'. If you play your part and do what is asked of you as a human being and member of a particular religion or of society, help will come in some way or another. A good way to receive blessings and help and assistance is through prayers and petitions and also a Goals list, which is mentioned in many personal development materials.

There is a saying, 'Goals not Gifts' are better for a person. Goals are like prayers and petitions, but written down, and the visual senses are the most powerful sensory organ for most people; seeing what you have written as well as hearing what you have written is very powerful for learning and structuring your environment in your favour.

It is how the world and spiritual world will respond to you when you start planning and moulding your environment to how you need and want. For example, if you are in a shopping centre car park and you start to look for a parking space, the environment will respond with cars reversing out and people walking to their cars with their shopping.

9. Sin

In Christianity, some people confuse the element of Sin. Yes we are Sinners, but that does not mean we purposely go chase the Sin. Ok you are a Christian, Jesus came for the Sinners, go and sin. However, some people do this. The reality is aiming to live a good life and sin will come your way from time-to-time. Otherwise people would be getting sick, injured and possibly dying more often from ill-treating themselves through Sin. Yet, we see stories in the news all the time about what has happened next in the private and public lives of people locally and around the world.

The key for Sinners is repentance, through the Church or place of worship and religion and personally with the Lord or God, and trying not to sin again. The Catholic Church has confession for Sinners, but some other Christian denominations do not have Reconciliation (confession), let alone Communion/Eucharist, and are just Bible based. Yet the Lord still loves them and wants them to repent and come back to him – Hymn: 'Come Back to Me (with all your heart)'.

How to combat sin is to have spiritual and religious and worldly strategies in place. There is the Mass or Worship, Prayers, Good Deeds and Charity; and Healing and Deliverance from a spiritual and religious viewpoint. Then there are things such as Health; Work and Education; Hobbies and Interests and Relationships and Socialising on a worldly level.

10. Heaven, a better place and End-of-world talk

Most people are good people, and most of us want to go to a better place. However, some people might be educated differently, are ignorant or have been associating with the wrong company to have this belief be tarnished or negatively turned around.

It is true we will all face death at some stage. So whether we like it or not, we will experience the eternal realm after death. Some people are ready, others somewhat or not at all. If you were to die today, where would you go do you think?

Some people think Heaven is on Earth, and this is true to a large extent. People in general have some freedom to live their lives, as life is short, and then pass away and enter the eternal realm. However, some people believe Heaven should be on Earth; in other words we will return again to the Earth to live our lives in our spiritual-human bodies. This can well happen, but then again, what about Heaven after death, in the spiritual eternal realm? Where does that fit in?

One can possibly state that we as a people can live here on Earth and venture between Heaven in the eternal realm as well as Heaven on Earth. Or, when we are ready, we can return to Heaven in the eternal realm.

The end of the world can mean different things to different people. Most people, I'm sure, would want to finish off safely and properly. However, some would want an almost over-the-top dramatical exit. The latter point is honestly a bit dangerous because innocent and good people could get caught in these dramatists workings. Some religions speak of this latter dramatical ending-of-the-world, but is there really a need for it? This world and society took a lot of effort to be where it is today, going through changes and developments to earn our freedom, for example WWI and WWII. Surely some of this world and society is kept in Heaven in the eternal realm, and good parts of Hell. Maybe that is just it; people want to keep and preserve this way of life here on Earth, at least to some extent.

Such a dramatical end-of-the-world fits in with the workings of the Devil. The Devil likes disharmony and discontent, which is what this dramatical end-of-the-world is. My advice is to just ignore it and have no part in it and to keep one's focus on that better place in Heaven.

The Physicality of the eternal realm, when used constructively, and from a Christian viewpoint, involves your Baptismal spirit assigned to you, the Lord Jesus, the Holy Spirit, the Trinity and certain Angels and Saints that pass through you at certain times of your worldly and spiritual existence. These spiritual entities will help and assist you to get through your life here on Earth and in Heaven and eternal life.

11. Rituals and Procedures in a Religion

Most religions have its own rituals and procedures to make it what it is. Some practitioners know it, others do not know it as much. Then again, there are people who are complex and those who are simpler, and combinations of this, and this needs to be respected.

If a person is new to a religion, or has not practiced often, they will lack the knowledge and understanding of someone who has been in the religion for a while. An example is going for Communion/ Eucharist in the Catholic-Christian Church. Usually a person who has not been to Communion/Eucharist for a while needs to go to Confession/Reconciliation to repent for their sins before going to Communion/Eucharist. But some people who come into the Church do not go to confession and go straight to Communion unclean. Now a person who has been going to Church for a while would know this, and a person who had not, would not know. It is up to these long-serving parishioners or the Priest or Pastor to remind these other people of this.

Some people find religion or Church or a place of worship to be boring or unstimulating, hence the growth of Churches like Hillsong. These Churches do have a positive vibe about them and do have the Bible and Pastors speaking about all different topics. However, there is a lack of spirituality and solemness in such Churches. Some of these people who attend Hillsong or similar Churches lack that true and deeper understanding of why they go to Church.

In stating this, the mass, along with the Eucharist/Communion, and Confession/Repentance, are powerful sacraments and are prayers and healing in themselves. The same goes in other religions and their practices.

For example, Angels appeared in the Church to the husband of a wife who had been trying for many years to bring him to Church. He changed, and began to attend Church, help others and speak occasionally to the congregation of the Church. One thing a person can say when attending a Church or place of worship, is 'Angels in the Church/Place of Worship, please help me'.

12. Literature in religion

Reading and listening to spiritual or religious information, along with all what encompasses a religion, can provide positivity, foundation, hope, love, motivation and enthusiasm and structure, amongst other things. Some good Pastors are Joyce Meyer, Joel Osteen and David Jeremiah, who are all on YouTube or have material one can purchase.

A person may be simpler and read less, another individual may be complex and read more. When reading important and Holy publications and material in a religion, such as the Holy Bible in Christianity, it is best to take a structured, educated and cautious approach to taking in such information. For example, just opening the Holy Bible at any page leaves this approach open to reading and taking in ill-proper and incorrect information. A person should either use a study guide or have the spiritual leader or participant, such as a Priest or Pastor, select some relevant and appropriate lines and passages to read and consume.

Like rituals and procedures in a religion, both types of person, simple and complex, should be respected. However, for the simple person, not being informed, and having some strong basis and foundation, is dangerous in this day-in-age as they can be misled and or deceived. One should have some wisdom and knowledge about their faith and life in general, at least.

However, one should not cut off the world's information on life as life can be someone's best teacher, for example, personal development material. One does not sit a course or education in their house or place of worship, it is done in society. In stating this, a blend of worldly and spiritual and religious material should be used to help and motivate your life. One should be careful and cautious though what wisdom, knowledge and information they take in and this depends on the person, group, culture and religion.

Bibliography

- Personal experiences:
    - I thought about being a Life Coach at one stage, but decided to make my own areas of life that needed to be concentrated on, including Faith (Also Health, Activities and Relationships).

    - I personally being 'in the spirit', with my blend of worldly and spiritual knowledge having progressed so far.

www.ingramcontent.com/pod-product-compliance
Lightning Source LLC
Chambersburg PA
CBHW081800280526
45789CB00008B/2940